A Commonsense
Guide to Fasting

A Commonsense Guide to Fasting

Kenneth E. Hagin

18 17 16 15 14 13 12 11   31 30 29 28 27 26 25 24

A Commonsense Guide to Fasting
ISBN-13: 978-0-89276-403-7
ISBN-10: 0-89276-403-1

In the U.S. write:
Kenneth Hagin Ministries
P.O. Box 50126
Tulsa, OK 74150-0126
1-888-28-FAITH
www.rhema.org

In Canada write:
Kenneth Hagin Ministries of Canada
P.O. Box 335, Station D
Etobicoke (Toronto), Ontario
Canada M9A 4X3
1-866-70-RHEMA
www.rhemacanada.org

CONTENTS

PREFACE

In all the Epistles—the books of the New Testament written to the Church—not one time is the Church told to fast.

That doesn't mean we should not. Mention is made of fasting, but no rules are laid down, nor is the Church even encouraged to fast.

The reason is, fasting is to be done as the occasion arises.

Fasting does not change God. He is the same before, during, and after you fast.

But fasting will change you. It will help you keep the flesh under. It will help you become more sensitive to the Spirit of God.

It is good to fast when things are pressing in upon you and you need to wait on God prayerfully. Or, the Lord may speak to you and lead you to fast. If the Lord lays a fast on your heart, do it! He has spoken to me in this manner several times. The longest I have ever fasted, however, is three days.

The Bible lists these reasons for fasting:

1. To minister to the Lord.
2. To lay hands on ministers to send them forth.
3. To draw close to God in times of danger.

These are the scriptural reasons; you don't need to fast to defeat the devil. Jesus already won that victory for us.

Remembering this, we can use fasting sensibly to keep the body under. The following pages will show the scriptural basis for this commonsense approach to fasting.

1

Fasting: A Look at the Old Testament

Fasting has in all ages and among all nations been an exercise much in use in times of mourning, sorrow, and afflictions.

Yet there is no Bible example of fasting to be seen before the time of Moses. Although the Bible doesn't say so, it is presumed that the patriarchs of old fasted until Moses' time. (We know this because there was a great deal of mourning among people of the Old Covenant.)

It is interesting to notice that Moses enjoined no particular fast in his five books, except upon the solemn Day of Atonement. In Leviticus 23:27, Moses talks about "afflicting your souls." In Hebrew this means, "Ye shall humble yourself deeply before God inwardly by sorrow, and by judging and loathing yourselves; and outwardly by fasting and abstinence from all carnal comforts and delights."

This fast is the *only* one Moses enjoins, although the Jews did fast at other times for periods of 24 hours: from the sundown of one day to the sundown of the next.

Since the time of Moses, examples of fasting have been common among the Jews. After Israel's defeat at Ai, Joshua and the leaders lay on their faces before God until evening (Josh. 7:6). In other words, it was from morning until evening; about 12 hours.

Judges 20:26 speaks of fasting until evening, and First Samuel 7:6 and Second Samuel 12:16 also give examples of fasting.

Should My Goal Be a 40-Day Fast?

A mistake many people make in teaching on fasting is picking out isolated portions of Scripture and misconstruing them. Any Bible subject can be pushed out of context and do more harm than good.

Some writers leave the impression everyone should go on a 40-day fast. They use the illustration that Moses fasted 40 days on Mount Horeb.

But consider this: Moses was in the very presence of God. If you were on a mountain in the presence of God, talking to Him, you probably could go without food and water 40 days, too!

Exodus 34:28 says, *"And he was there with the Lord forty days and forty nights; he did neither eat bread, nor drink water. And he wrote upon the tables the words of the covenant, the ten commandments."*

The Scripture prior to this says God appeared to him. The glory of God was there, and Moses was caught up in it. He could well go without food or water.

Nobody can go without water very long unless he is in a supernatural condition. You can go without food, but not water.

If you're caught up in the Spirit and are in the glory of God, you also lose all sense of time. Those 40 days probably seemed like about 14 minutes to Moses.

Sister Maria Woodworth-Etter, one of the pioneers of the Pentecostal movement, was still preaching in a tent that would seat 20,000 when she was 72 years old. She would fill it up and preach without a public address system. When she ministered, the power of God often came upon her as well as upon others in the congregation.

For example, in one of Sister Etter's books she reports that during a tent revival in Shawnee, Ohio, the Spirit of God came upon a woman and the woman lay under the power of God for eight days. During that time she did not take any nourishment. At the end of that time, she came up shouting and preaching, telling others of the wonderful experience she had had. Naturally, anyone caught up in such glory could go without food, water, or anything else. (*A Diary of Signs and Wonders*, Etter, p. 107.)

Some say Elijah fasted 40 days, but actually he didn't. Jezebel threatened to cut his head off, so he ran. Wearily, he climbed under a juniper tree and cried, "Just let me die. I would just as soon be dead!" But he didn't want to die any more than you would if you had said that. If he had really wanted to die, he could have stayed where he was—Jezebel would have accommodated him!

The Lord came and ministered to him, and the angels fed him. He went in the strength of that angel food 40 days. First Kings 19:7 says, *"And the angel of the Lord came again the second time, and touched him, and said, Arise and eat; because the journey is too great for thee."*

If an angel came down and fed you, you might be able to go in the strength of that quite a while, too. But that's not a *bona fide* fast. You can't use that as an example of someone fasting in the natural.

The only one whom the Bible ever said fasted 40 days was Jesus. In Matthew 4:2 we read, *"And when he had fasted forty days and forty nights, he was afterward an hungered."* There is a clue here. Matthew 4:1 says he was *"led up of the spirit into the wilderness to be tempted of the devil."* So He was led by the Spirit and ministered to by angels. Again, that's not a *bona fide* fast.

2

Fasting: A Look at the New Testament

Nowhere in the New Testament did Jesus institute any kind of fast. In His commands to His disciples, Jesus never enjoined any fast to be kept.

Paul said he fasted, but in all his letters to the Church, starting with Romans, *there is not a single reference telling the Church to fast.* We're encouraged to pray, but in connection with demon activity, healing, or anything else, we are not told to fast.

Fasting, then, must not be as important as some people would lead you to believe. There would have to be some kind of instruction to the Church if it were! There are instructions on the gifts of the Spirit, praying, and giving, but none on fasting.

Let's go to the four Gospels and look at some things Jesus said about fasting.

LUKE 5:33-35

33 And they said unto him, Why do the disciples of John fast often, and make prayers, and likewise the disciples of the Pharisees; but thine eat and drink?

34 And he said unto them, Can ye make the children of the bridechamber fast, while the bridegroom is with them?

35 But the days will come, when the bridegroom shall be taken away from them, and then shall they fast in those days.

At one point Jesus did leave the disciples, but He did come back, and He's with us today.

"Appear Not Unto Men to Fast"

We read in Matthew 6 something else Jesus said about fasting:

MATTHEW 6:16-18

16 Moreover when ye fast, be not, as the hypocrites, of a sad countenance: for they disfigure their faces, that they may appear unto men to fast. Verily I say unto you, They have their reward.

17 But thou, when thou fastest, anoint thine head, and wash thy face;

18 That thou appear not unto men to fast, but unto thy Father which is in secret: and thy Father, which seeth in secret, shall reward thee openly.

In my opinion, a person who talks about how long he fasts and encourages others to fast a long time is a hypocrite.

I held a meeting once for a man and his wife. The pastor's wife was also a minister. She got up every night and said something like," I'm on the fifth day of my fast. I wonder if there are those who will join me?"

It would have helped just as much if she had twiddled her thumbs and said, "I'm on the fifth day of twiddling my thumbs." As far as God was concerned, she had lost all her reward. Even though I was fasting, I never publicly joined her, because I didn't want to appear unto men to fast.

There may be certain occasions when you would solicit the church to fast as the Lord would lead you. But what she was doing was getting up and bragging every night about herself.

If we go around bragging about how much we pray and how long we fast, that's not good. Jesus said not to appear unto men to fast. To me, that would mean don't let them know it. Do it as unto God, your Father, in secret. And your Father who sees in secret will reward you openly.

Fasting in the Book of Acts

The Word of God mentions fasting again in Acts; nevertheless, there is no direction given to the Church on when to fast. The Bible says in Acts 10 that Cornelius was fasting.

He wasn't even saved at this time. But being a Jewish proselyte, he naturally fasted because the Jews did.

ACTS 10:30

30 And Cornelius said, Four days ago I was fasting until this hour, and at the ninth hour I prayed in my house, and behold, a man stood before me in bright clothing....

That was an angel, of course, who told him to send for Peter in Joppa to come and preach to them. Since Cornelius was a Jewish proselyte, we can't count that as a reference to members of the Church fasting. He wasn't saved until Peter came.

As I studied this, I was amazed at how little fasting is mentioned in the Bible. We do have further references in Acts 13 and 14.

Acts 14:23 says, *"And when they had ordained them elders in every church, and had prayed with fasting, they commended them to the Lord, on whom they believed."*

Here elders were being ordained.

It's good for people to fast and miss one meal. It is a good thing to fast before you pray for the sick. But it doesn't mean the apostles went on a long fast.

In Acts 13 something similar happened. In the first verse, five prophets and teachers are mentioned. Among them were Saul (Paul), and Barnabas. As these five men ministered to the Lord and fasted, the Holy Spirit said,

"Separate me Barnabas and Saul for the work whereunto I have called them" (v. 2).

Verse 3 says: *"And when they had fasted and prayed. . . ."* They already mentioned they were ministering to the Lord and fasting. We read this as though the two incidents happened together. But evidently that is not true, because it takes time to fast again. It says, *"And when they had fasted and prayed and laid their hands on them. . . ."*

This probably took place over a period of time. They took some time to wait on God. Again, fasting didn't change God. But it did help them become more sensitive to the Holy Spirit.

Did you know spiritualists fast? They are in contact with demons and evil spirits, and they believe fasting helps them become more sensitive to *evil spirits.* That is the reason the devil gets to working on some people when they start fasting—especially when they try to fast for long periods of time. You've got to realize there are many spirits in the spirit world.

We find two other references to fasting in Acts chapter 27. *"Now when much time was spent, and when sailing was now dangerous, because the fast was now already past, Paul admonished them . . ."* (Acts 27:9). When Paul says the fast was over and sailing was dangerous, he is referring to the tenth day of the seventh month—the time of Atonement— which was a time of fasting.

Many Jews in the Early Church, even though they were born again and Spirit filled, still kept the traditions of the Jewish religion. Prayer was more of a struggle under the Old Covenant, because Jesus hadn't come and conquered the devil.

In the 33rd and 34th verses of that same chapter it says, *"And while the day was coming on, Paul besought them all to take meat, saying, This is the fourteenth day that ye have tarried and continued fasting, having taken nothing. Wherefore I pray you to take some meat: for this is for your health: for there shall not an hair fall from the head of any of you."*

Often the Bible uses the word "meat" to stand for food. The ship had sailed and weathered a storm, and Paul was inferring he didn't want them to go too long without food. He said, "This is for your health."

Verse 35 says, *"And when he had thus spoken, he took bread, and gave thanks to God in presence of them all: and when he had broken it, he began to eat."* An angel of the Lord had appeared to him and told him they were all going to be saved.

I repeat: There are no instructions given to the Church to tell them to fast or not to fast. The records we have in Acts show that the apostles ministered to the Lord and fasted, and it seems the Lord would be pleased if we would set aside some time just to minister to Him.

If you fast and don't minister to the Lord, it might not do you too much good. But fasting will give you that extra time to wait on God. At the same time, it will help you keep the flesh under.

You Must Have a Purpose

As mentioned before, it seems in the New Testament that people fasted under these conditions: to minister to the Lord, to ordain men to the ministry, or to seek God in times of extreme danger. You always must have a purpose. Don't fast just because someone tells you to.

Don't Fast for Revival

I've known some pastors who try to fast for a revival. But as Charles G. Finney said, a revival is no more miraculous than a farmer's reaping a crop. The farmer has to till the ground, plant the seed, cultivate, and trust God to send the rain. (I know we have irrigation these days, but we still need rain in the first place.)

Remember that Paul, in writing to the Church at Corinth, said: *"I have planted, Apollos watered; but God gave the increase"* (I Cor. 3:6). You can fast until doomsday that God will save souls, but if you don't get out there and witness to people, preach salvation, and "go into all the world and preach the Gospel to every creature," nobody will get saved—and I don't care how long you fast.

Nowhere in Scripture did they fast for a revival. Nowhere did they fast for a mighty move of God.

What did they do? First, they ministered to the Lord. They weren't praying they'd get something; they just wanted to take time to visit with the Lord.

I'm sure they ministered to Him like the Bible said: *"Be not drunk with wine wherein is excess; but be filled with the Spirit; Speaking to yourselves in psalms and hymns and spiritual songs, singing and making melody in your heart to the Lord"* (Eph. 5:18,19).

When I was in revival meetings I'd spend the whole day (we didn't have day services in some of the churches) in the church building. I would be walking up and down the aisle, reading my Bible around the altar, praying, and ministering to the Lord. I just set that time aside to minister to the Lord.

Second, they fasted in Bible times to lay hands on ministers to send them forth. And third, they fasted in times of extreme danger. If I had an emergency come up, I would begin to fast and pray to get an answer. I never fasted as long as three full days, because I always got my answer. I took extra time to wait on God, to pray, and the answer would come in various ways. If I had a spiritual question, for example, I would get the revelation.

(3)

Why Doesn't Paul
Tell Us to Fast?

Again, there are no instructions telling the Church to fast.

Paul, in writing to the Church at Corinth, makes reference to the fact that he fasted, although he doesn't encourage the Corinthians to fast or give them any direction about it. He says:

2 CORINTHIANS 6:4,5

4 But in all things approving ourselves as the ministers of God, in much patience, in afflictions, in necessities, in distresses,

5 In stripes, in imprisonments, in tumults, in labours, in watchings, in fastings.

So we know Paul did fast.

Yet he didn't tell the Church to fast. Some say, "But don't we need to fast to get power over the devil?" Jesus Himself said in the 17th chapter of Matthew about evil spirits that *"this kind goeth not out but by prayer and fasting."*

Yes, He said that. But, you see, Jesus hadn't died yet. When He died and was raised to newness of life, He soundly defeated the devil and all his cohorts. Jesus has whipped the devil!

In First Corinthians we're told these powers are dethroned powers. Jesus said, *"IN MY NAME shall they cast out devils"* (Mark 16:17). You don't have to fast to get the Name of Jesus. Fasting has no part in casting out devils except that it will help you become more sensitive to the Spirit of God. It will help you keep the flesh under.

That's why the Epistles don't tell us anything in this area. Jesus said, after He arose from the dead, *"Go ye into all the world, and preach the gospel"* (Mark 16:15). He said to tell the Good News; tell people you're delivered from sin. He's already done it: He's cancelled all our sins, and He has defeated the devil.

Remember, *"Ye are of God, little children, and have overcome them: because greater is he that is in you, than he that is in the world"* (1 John 4:4). He was your Substitute. What He did is marked up to your credit.

No wonder Paul wouldn't give instructions to the Church on fasting. *As an aid to putting the flesh under, fasting has a real purpose; but as to conquering the devil and sin, Jesus has already done it, and we are in Him!*

In Ephesians, we are told we have been quickened together with Christ:

EPHESIANS 2:2-5

2 Wherein in time past ye walked according to the course of this world, according to the prince of the power of the air, the spirit that now worketh in the children of disobedience:

3 Among whom also we all had our conversation in times past in the lusts of our flesh, fulfilling the desires of the flesh and of the mind; and were by nature the children of wrath, even as others.

4 But God, who is rich in mercy, for his great love wherewith he loved us,

5 Even when we were dead in sins, hath quickened us together with Christ.

Can you see that? Jesus was our Substitute. In Colossians 2:15 it says He spoiled principalities and powers. Those are the same principalities and powers we wrestle with in Ephesians 6:12—and He made a show of them openly, triumphing over them in it. Jesus won a real victory, and we won that victory with Him.

So, *you* have overcome them. The Bible doesn't say, "If you'll fast 14 days you'll overcome them." No, you've got a right to use the Name of Jesus! That Name belongs to you *whether you fast or not.* And in Jesus' Name you've got a right to exercise authority over demons.

Paul, in writing to the Church at Ephesus, said, *"Neither give place to the devil"* (Eph. 4:27). He didn't say, "Now if you'll fast for a week or two or fast three or four days. . . ." The devil might take over while you are trying to get in a position to do something. He said not to give the devil any place in you. That means he can't take a place unless you let him.

James said, *"Resist the devil, and he will flee from you"* (James 4:7). *You* do it. You'd have to have the authority over him or you couldn't do it!

What did Peter say? *"Be sober, be vigilant; because your adversary the devil, as a roaring lion, walketh about, seeking whom he may devour"* (1 Peter 5:8). What are you going to do about it? Resist him! Stand steadfast in the faith.

Fasting and
Self-Control

There is something else the New Testament says:

1 CORINTHIANS 7:4,5

4 The wife hath not power of her own body, but the husband: and likewise also the husband hath not power of his own body, but the wife.

5 Defraud ye not one the other, except it be with consent for a time, that ye may give yourselves to FASTING AND PRAYER; and come together again, that Satan tempt you not for your incontinency.

Another translation says not to withhold sexual intercourse from one another, except it be with consent, that you may give yourselves to *fasting and prayer.* This is the only reference to fasting and prayer mentioned in the letters written to the Church; yet notice no particular fast is instituted here. We are only made aware that people did fast and pray.

Paul said, "And come together again," talking about husband and wife coming together so Satan couldn't tempt them "for your incontinency." That's plain enough, isn't it?

Here's something else about self-control and fasting. From 1949 through the late '50s, I'd stay in parsonages when I was traveling in the field ministry, and I noticed something—The pastors who shouted and hollered the most in the church *lived the worst* and fasted the least at home.

In keeping a record for three or four years I never could find one of them who could control his emotions.

One fellow I knew could holler the loudest, jump the highest, and make the most noise of anyone when he was in the pulpit. He actually said to me, "I can't miss a meal. I just can't do it." He would get upset when his wife didn't have dinner on the table on time.

I couldn't enjoy his shouting to save my life. I don't know whether he just got worked up physically or what, but I doubt if the Spirit of God had very much to do with it. He was living in the flesh. (Now, there is a real move of the Spirit, but some have never learned the difference between working something up and that real move that's so sweet and beautiful.)

I followed my procedure of fasting while I was with these folks. Naturally, they would invite me to come to the table to eat. I wouldn't say I was fasting, but I'd say, "I'm just not eating today. I want to spend a little time praying."

5

Fasting in My Life

When I was pastor of a Full Gospel church in East Texas, I was preparing to go one fall to a Bible conference. The Spirit of God said to me, "Fast the next two days, because they're going to ask you to pray for the sick at the meeting."

I laughed and said, "Why, dear Lord, if they do that, it'll be a real switch, because they've got hundreds of preachers. They've never asked me to pray or testify, much less pray for the sick. That couldn't be right."

Then I got to thinking about it. I knew I didn't think that up myself. I didn't really want to fast. (Sometimes we ask, "Can that be God? Is it the devil? Just who is talking to me?" We've got to learn to evaluate these things.)

I knew it couldn't be the flesh, because the flesh doesn't want to fast. And it couldn't be the devil. The devil wouldn't encourage you to fast in moderation; however, he might encourage you to go too far and break your body down.

(I know of a pastor who went on a long fast, didn't drink any water, broke his body down, and died as a result of it. His idea of fasting was entirely wrong. He thought he was going to move God.)

You're not going to move God. He doesn't move. He's already prone to do certain things, and He's going to do them just as soon as you get in contact with Him and let Him.

The next day I went to the Bible conference. As I sat down, the presbyter was speaking and was ready to turn the meeting over to the district superintendent. It was in their hands to do the preaching that morning.

The presbyter said, "I saw Brother Hagin come in and I didn't ask anybody, but the Lord has been dealing with me to have him hold a healing service tonight. We don't want to intrude on any of the services, so we'll start early. We'll give him at least an hour or more to minister to the sick."

That's the same thing the Spirit had said to me 120 miles away. "Fast the next two days because they're going to ask you to minister to the sick at the Bible conference."

The Lord did manifest Himself through me. Fasting made me more sensitive. It didn't change God; God was in the healing business *before* I fasted, *while I* was fasting, and *after* I got through fasting. It didn't prepare God any—it prepared me. It helped my spirit become more sensitive to His Spirit so His Spirit could manifest Himself through me.

The Fasted Life

When I first went out in the field ministry, I set aside two days a week—Tuesday and Thursday—for my fast days. I wasn't led of the Lord to do it; I just fasted two days a week. I fasted 24 hours, because that was the way Israel did it.

I took the extra time that I would have been eating to pray. Remember, fasting will not do you much good if you're not going to spend extra time praying, waiting on God.

I made the greatest spiritual strides yet in my ministry during that time of fasting two days a week. I shut myself up in my church and spent many hours praying.

I said to my wife, "I know when we eat. If I don't come out to eat, don't send the children after me. You'll know I'm going to skip that meal." I did quite a bit of fasting. I also did quite a bit of praying, and I spent that extra time in the Word of God. And often—because the church was next door—I got up and went over in the night to pray while everyone else was asleep.

One night I prayed all night long. Many nights I prayed *nearly* all night long. I spent time fellowshipping with God, waiting on Him, walking up and down the aisles praying. (There was enough light from the streetlight shining through the windows that I didn't have to turn the lights on.)

It wasn't just the fasting; it was the extra time I took to wait on God and spend time in His Word that did something for me spiritually. Fasting will help keep the flesh under and make you more sensitive to the Holy Spirit.

Singers know this principle. If they eat a big meal and try to come out and sing, they are bogged down. Preachers know that. That's the reason we don't like to eat before we preach. If we do, we find we are uncomfortable and not so spiritually sensitive.

After several years of fasting two days a week, the Lord said to me, "I would be more pleased if you would live a *fasted life.* I said, "What do you mean, a *fasted life?*"

He said, "Never eat all you want. Keep your appetite under. That's all a fast is going to do anyway; keep the body under."

Do you know that is harder than fasting? I changed. I never had any more *days* of fasting. I never set any times of fasting unless the Spirit of God spoke to me. And I made greater spiritual strides living *the fasted life.* Much of the time I ate only one meal a day while I was in meetings. (I still do that much of the time.)

I noticed that healings came more easily when I did this. When it came to laying hands on people to receive the Holy Spirit, I wouldn't eat at all. If we'd run into a hard spot and things weren't happening like I thought they should, I'd fast by drinking a little juice. If I needed more strength physically, I'd start eating, but I never ate all I wanted. I started having more results because I more or less constantly lived the fasted life.

One time I went to Kansas City to hold a meeting. When I got there, the pastor said, "Brother Hagin, something has arisen and I've got to be out of town part of this week. You go ahead and run the meeting to suit you and I'll be back toward the end of the week."

I preached Sunday night. Monday morning we had a Bible lesson at 10 a.m. Monday night I preached. Tuesday morning I preached (I usually carried two services a day). Tuesday night I preached. This was the third day.

One of the deacons said to me, "Brother Hagin, how do you like the restaurant at the motel?"

I stopped and said, "You know what? I never thought about it. I haven't eaten since I've been here. I forgot it."

Then I said, "That restaurant is closed down. There is a sign there that says 'Closed.'"

He said, "Oh, we intended for you to eat there. What have you been doing about eating?"

I said, "I never thought about eating until you mentioned it."

When he said something about eating, I got hungry. Until then, I had been so taken up with spiritual things I hadn't thought anything about it. (Incidentally, I ate every day from then on.)

For three weeks of meetings, those were the only three days I didn't eat. I wasn't fasting; I just never thought about eating. It never dawned on me to eat. When I did begin eating, I still had just one meal a day. What I'm trying to say is there are no iron-clad rules.

6

Pushing to Extremes

Don't be like the pastor who broke down his body with fasting and became so sick he died. The poor fellow suffered so. He was a wonderful man, but nobody could help him, because he wouldn't listen. You see, your body is still mortal. It hasn't been redeemed yet, and you are going to have to learn to take care of it. I learned that lesson early.

When I first started preaching, I didn't have the baptism of the Holy Spirit, but I did believe in divine healing. I was pastor of a little church in the country and had an extra job on the side.

One day I was working outdoors and knew I was getting too hot. I knew I ought to stop. Something on the inside of me—the inward witness—told me, but I didn't listen to it. I went right on, and had a heat stroke. My heart stopped, and I nearly died. I had Full Gospel people lay hands on me and pray for me, even though I was a Baptist.

You know, I couldn't get a thing until I repented and said, "Dear God, I repent. I'll never push my body to that place again." The minute I made that promise to God, I rose up perfectly healed.

Since that time I have refused to push myself to that extreme. I've been right in the middle of a healing line, realized I was physically getting to that place, and stopped and walked off. I've told the people I can't violate my conscience and break my contract with God.

Someone might say, "We'll just pray God will give you supernatural strength." Some people have the craziest ideas about these things; they believe you ought to be a superhuman.

Did you ever notice Jesus again and again departed from the crowd? His body was also flesh, blood, and bone. He got just as tired as anybody did. The main thing in all the affairs of life is to be led by the Spirit of God.

Some people try to make a religion out of fasting. They push themselves to an extreme, thinking *works* will get the job done. But I don't believe in *religion;* I believe in *Christ* and life in Christ. Don't get involved in works.

Let the Lord lead you. Take some time to fast and wait on God *as the Spirit of God leads you.* Feel free to obey Him.

I went to one place to hold revival, and we had the greatest revival in the history of that church. Sunday School doubled and church membership tripled. The pastor said night after night, "Boys, I just marvel at God moving in such a way. And we haven't even fasted."

He was trying to put it back on works; he thought works would get the job done. But I went believing God. God honors faith. That's the thing God honors more than anything else.

(7)

Different Kinds of Fasts

Remember how Daniel fasted 21 days? He ate no "pleasant bread." We need to realize there is more than one way to fast. Daniel didn't eat anything he wanted, but he did eat a little something. That is harder to do sometimes.

You see, it's a matter of keeping the flesh under; keeping the body under and not letting it dominate you. You dominate it instead.

If you wanted to go a step further, you could fast things other than food. You might say, "Now, Lord, I'm going to leave off watching television and spend that time praying." (Daniel said he gave up eating *pleasant bread*. So why wouldn't it be all right to leave off other things that might be pleasant to us?)

A well-known evangelist when he was pastoring decided to give God 10 percent of his time in prayer. He began to pray at night after his family was in bed. He prayed two hours and 40 minutes each night. To do that he had to sacrifice his television time. God has given him an internationally known ministry.

You might say, "I couldn't pray two hours and 40 minutes a day." But perhaps you could sacrifice television time, too, or some other time that you're wasting in order to devote more time to prayer.

(8)

What Can
I Accomplish
by Fasting?

Ministering to the Lord

The Bible gives us examples of people fasting to minister to the Lord. They weren't praying they'd get something; they just wanted to take some time to visit with the Lord.

ACTS 13:2,3

2 As they ministered to the Lord, and fasted, the Holy Ghost said, Separate me Barnabas and Saul for the work whereunto I have called them.

3 And when they had fasted and prayed, and laid their hands on them, they sent them away.

You might ask, "Now what do you mean, *ministered* to the Lord?" Well, I'm sure they prayed. But the Bible also says in Ephesians 5:18,19, *"And be not drunk with wine, wherein is excess; but be filled with the Spirit; Speaking*

*to yourselves in psalms and hymns and spiritual songs,
singing and making melody in your heart to the Lord."* They
began worshipping God and magnifying His name, and
went right through the meal!

Sometimes I'll speak to myself all night in psalms. I'm
ministering to the Lord. I've done that on more than one
occasion. A psalm is a spiritual poem or ode. It may or may
not rhyme, but there is an element of poetry in it. I get to
going sometimes very quietly in the nighttime to myself,
and they just keep rolling out of me.

When the Bible talks about psalms and hymns and
spiritual songs, this doesn't mean songs you get out of
a songbook. Most of those are embalmed with unbelief.
They are not inspired by the Spirit of God. The Bible is
talking about something the Spirit of God gives you on the
spur of the moment by the Holy Spirit.

We have 150 psalms in the Old Testament that were
given by the Spirit of God. They bless us because they are
Spirit anointed. Many of David's psalms were given to him
while he was going through tests or trials. They were his;
they blessed him; they encouraged him. A psalm can be
recited or chanted. The Jews chanted some of them.

A spiritual song or hymn was always sung. I seldom
sing, except in tongues, because I'm not a singer. (Paul

said, "I will pray in the spirit and I'll sing in the spirit"; that is, in tongues.) I usually speak in psalms. Buddy Harrison, my son-in-law, sings spiritual songs and hymns; something that the Spirit of God gives him at the moment.

Ministering to the Lord is worshipping Him; not wanting anything. We ought to have services in our churches where we minister to the Lord. If I were pastor of a church, I would have services once a week that I would call "believers' meetings." Nobody but believers would come, and we would minister to the Lord.

In one church I pastored, we usually had just our own people in the Sunday morning service. Sunday night was our evangelistic service. We filled the building at night. People would even be out on the street looking in through the doors. But Sunday mornings we rarely had nonmembers, so I made that Sunday morning service a believers' meeting.

I don't suppose I preached half a dozen times on Sunday morning from 1939 to 1940. I said to the people, "I'm going to sit down here on the platform and turn the service over to the Holy Spirit. Whatever you feel led of God to do, do it. If you feel led to start a chorus, just start singing."

I think we got the closest to what Paul was talking about at Corinth when he said,

I CORINTHIANS 14:26

26 How is it then, brethren? when ye come together, every one of you hath a psalm, hath a doctrine, hath a tongue, hath a revelation, hath an interpretation. Let all things be done unto edifying.

They went to church because they *had* something. But now most folks go to church to *get* something.

We had some of the most tremendous services. I've never seen anything like them before or since. And I'm convinced God wants that in every church. But we get so taken up with our little form. We think we have to be out by noon.

Sometimes in these meetings we would stay until 1:30 p.m. Sometimes the presence of God would move in on us and we would all just sit there. Not a child cried. Nobody moved. Nobody would say anything. We sat there sometimes 45 minutes. The power of God—the presence of God—was so real you didn't want to move. You were afraid if you moved a finger, the presence would go away.

One fellow would bring his wife, who was saved, to these services, and then he would go uptown to talk, chew, whittle, and cuss. One time he came back around noon, expecting the service to be over, but it wasn't. He sat in the car but didn't hear anything.

Finally he came inside. He felt what we were feeling the moment he walked in. Nobody said anything or turned to look at him. Since I was sitting on the platform, I could see him. He sat down, looked at me, and looked at the crowd. Nobody said anything; there was just a holy silence. I watched him because I knew something was going to happen.

He sat there about 10 minutes and suddenly began shaking all over. Then he got up and started down the aisle, still shaking, and fell at the altar. He started calling on God and got saved! Still, nobody said anything. No one went down to help him pray. God started it and finished it. He saved that fellow. I saw that happen more than once.

Sometimes the Spirit of God would move on somebody to start dancing. Before you knew it, 15 to 30 others would join him. They might dance all through the morning service. We charged that atmosphere with the Spirit of God.

I would tell the people, *"Now, when we come tonight, it's for a different purpose. We're not coming tonight to get blessed. We're not coming tonight to minister to the Lord. We are coming to reach the sinner. So be very careful that everything is done decently and in order"* (1 Cor. 14:40).

We had people saved, filled with the Holy Spirit, and healed every Sunday night. We had constant revival, because we kept that place charged with the power of God. In a lot of places the atmosphere is charged with deadness on Sunday morning. You need to get there early to expel all the demons the people bring in; otherwise, you fall flat on your face.

We need times of worship; times to worship any way the Lord leads us. That's what it means to minister unto the Lord.

Another reason they fasted in Bible times was to ordain men to the ministry or to separate them, as God would call them. I'm sure they didn't go on a long fast. They missed maybe one meal.

Facing Decisions and Times of Crisis

Many times in revival meetings when people seemed to have difficulty getting baptized with the Holy Spirit, I would tell them not to eat their evening meal. Without exception, it seemed to work easily; I've seen times when every one of them was filled with the Spirit.

You will find, too, as I've mentioned, that the Bible says in times of crisis men fasted.

Many times before Jesus made certain decisions, like selecting the apostles, He spent time apart.

Acts 27 is an example of Paul's fasting during a crisis. He was on his way by ship to appeal his case before Caesar and a storm arose.

ACTS 27:20

20 And when neither sun nor stars in many days appeared, and no small tempest lay on us, all hope that we should be saved was then taken away.

Paul had perceived danger by the Spirit of God before the voyage.

ACTS 27:21-25

21 But after long abstinence Paul stood forth in the midst of them, and said, Sirs, ye should have hearkened unto me, and not have loosed from Crete, and to have gained this harm and loss.

22 And now I exhort you to be of good cheer—for there shall be no loss of any man's life among you, but of the ship.

23 For there stood by me this night the angel of God, whose I am, and whom I serve,

24 Saying, Fear not, Paul; thou must be brought before Caesar: and, lo, God hath given thee all them that sail with thee.

25 Wherefore, sirs, be of good cheer: for I believe God, that it shall be even as it was told me.

I don't know how long Paul fasted here, but after abstaining from food he stood in their midst. He told the men their lives would be spared. He had abstained from food for some time and had sought God. In a letter to some of the churches concerning his own ministry he used the expression "in fastings often."

9

Setting Free
the Oppressed

There was a woman in a church we pastored who had a large tumor on her left lung. She had gone to her family doctor, but he sent her to a specialist in a larger city nearby. This was in 1939, and they didn't operate on people so quickly then.

They did not know whether the tumor was malignant or not, but they gave her X-ray treatments. They said the treatments wouldn't cure her, but they were supposed to retard the growth of the tumor or shrink it. If these treatments were unsuccessful, the next step was the operation, which in those days was very serious.

I knew she was taking these treatments twice a week, but she never asked for prayer.

On the day when she went to the city to take her treatment, her 16-year-old daughter was home (this was in the summer). They lived on a farm and had to get up early to go to the city; the trip took a full day. All that day, which was a Thursday, the 16-year-old girl fasted and prayed for her mother. She prayed that the oppressed might be set free. (Acts 10:38 speaks of sickness as being satanic oppression.)

I knew nothing about what had happened. When I closed my sermon the following Sunday morning, the voice of the Lord came to me saying, "There's a lady here I want to heal before you go today." So I spoke it right out without thinking. That's the first time a thing like that had happened. This was 1939. I spoke it right out, saying, "The Lord just said there's a woman here whom He wants to heal before we go today."

When I said that, a lady stepped out. She started down the aisle, but the Spirit of God within me said, "She's not the one."

I said, "Sister, you're not the one, but healing belongs to you, so come on and we'll pray for you, and the Lord will heal you."

Then Sister R. stepped out in the aisle and the Spirit of God within me said, "She's the one." I told her, "Sister R., you're the one." I laid hands on her and prayed and that tumor disappeared. She went back to the specialist and told him to take X-rays because something had happened. He asked, "What is it?" She replied, "I'll tell you afterwards."

He took the X-rays and couldn't find the tumor. He tried taking more, but still couldn't find it. It was gone.

I was holding a meeting in a Full Gospel church in Houston, Texas, a number of years ago, and I was staying in the parsonage. The pastor's wife never said one word to me about her poor physical condition. (She had prayed for years and never had received anything.)

God began to move in the services and bless people. Many were being healed. Afterwards, this pastor's wife testified, "I saw others being healed and I fasted." (She fixed something for her husband and me to eat, but she never sat down with us.)

"I fasted and prayed a couple of days," she said, "and told the Lord I knew He could heal me."

One night I was ministering after I preached, and I had a revelation concerning her. I began telling her what was wrong with her, because I saw it in the spirit; the Lord told me exactly what was wrong with her. The Word of Knowledge was in operation, and she received complete healing.

Although fasting in itself will not bring about healing, it can prepare the way in some instances for healing to take place.

(10)

A Final Word

Smith Wigglesworth said there were two young fellows in England who saw God's power demonstrated in his meetings at his wife's mission.

"We wouldn't be surprised but what God would lead you down to Wales to raise up our Lazarus," they told him.

They explained that Lazarus was a man who had spent his days working in a tin mine and his nights preaching. He had collapsed and become ill with tuberculosis, and for four years had been a helpless invalid, having to be fed with a spoon.

Two years later the Lord spoke to Wigglesworth. Often this great man of faith would walk in the countryside. One day he climbed one of the highest mountains in Wales. He was on top, enveloped in the presence of God, when the Lord said to him, "I want you to go raise Lazarus."

Wigglesworth wrote down what the Lord had said on a postcard, and mailed it to Lazarus' home. When he arrived, he was greeted at the door by a man holding the card. "Did you send this?" the man asked. "Do you think we believe in this? Here, take it!" And he threw it at Wigglesworth.

Then the man called a servant and said, "Take this man and show him Lazarus." He said to Wigglesworth, "The moment you see him, you will be ready to go home."

From the natural standpoint, this was true. The man was helpless. He was nothing but a mass of skin and bones—and he didn't have an ounce of faith.

Wigglesworth knew when God has spoken, you don't give in. He left, but overnight rounded up seven others to stand with him in prayer. That night the Spirit of the Lord told him not to eat, so he skipped the evening meal and skipped breakfast the following morning. (He believed prayer and fasting to be a great joy.)

The next day the eight of them went back to Lazarus' house. The same man let them in, and there lay that poor fellow looking like a corpse.

While Smith had been fasting, God had told him what to do: "Don't pray; don't anoint him with oil; don't touch him. All eight of you gather around the bed, hold hands, and repeat the Name of Jesus."

So he said, "We just stood around the bed and said, 'Jesus, Jesus, Jesus (all eight of them in unison), Jesus, Jesus!'"

As they spoke, the power of God fell. Then it lifted like a cloud. They continued to hold hands and say, "Jesus, Jesus" and the power kept coming down and lifting. The sixth time it came down Lazarus said, "I've been bitter in my heart, and I know I have grieved the Spirit of God." He repented and cried out, "O God, let this be to thy glory." As he said that, the power of God went through him, healing him.

Lazaurus got up and dressed himself without any assistance. Then he and Smith walked downstairs singing the Doxology. Lazarus testified in an open-air meeting what God had done and many were saved.

All the Spirit had said to Smith was, "Just miss two meals." That's all. Did that change God? No. God had already told him to raise up Lazarus. You see, it gave Wigglesworth *a little more time to wait on God instead of eating. It made his spirit more keen, and it made him more susceptible to God's Spirit so he could be a channel.*

That is why there are no instructions given by the Holy Spirit through Paul or Peter or James or John to fast or not to fast.

I believe this is because God wants us to learn to be led by His Spirit. That way we'll be prepared for whatever He has for us to do. Or, if the Spirit doesn't tell you to fast, set aside some time and say, "I am going to take this time to fast and wait on God and study my Bible."

When should you fast? I can't tell you, and the Bible doesn't give you specific instructions. That leaves it up to the leading of the Lord. The more you study, the more you can see how dependent we are on the Spirit of God; not only the Word of God, but the Holy Spirit.

No wonder Jesus said, "I'll not leave you comfortless." Another translation says "orphans." We need the help of the Holy Spirit—and we have it—in this area, as in all others.

Why should you consider attending
RHEMA
Bible Training Center?

Here are a few good reasons:

- Training at one of the top Spirit-filled Bible schools anywhere
- Teaching based on steadfast faith in God's Word
- Growth in your spiritual walk coupled with practical training in effective ministry
- Specialization in the area of your choosing: Youth or Children's Ministry, Evangelism, Pastoral Care, Missions, Biblical Studies, or Supportive Ministry
- Optional intensive third-year programs: School of Worship, School of Pastoral Ministry, School of World Missions, and General Extended Studies
- Worldwide ministry opportunities—while you're in school
- An established network of churches and ministries around the world who depend on RHEMA to supply full-time staff and support ministers
- A two-year evening school taught entirely in Spanish is also available. Log on to **www.cebrhema.org** for more information.

Call today for information or application material.
1-888-28-FAITH (1-888-283-2484)
www.rbtc.org

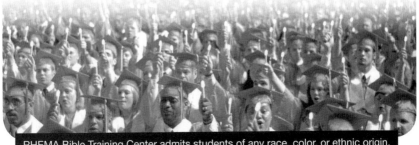

RHEMA Bible Training Center admits students of any race, color, or ethnic origin.

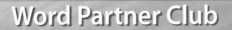

Word Partner Club

WORKING *together* TO REACH THE WORLD!

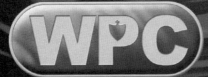

People. Power. Purpose.

Have you ever dropped a stone into water? Small waves rise up at the point of impact and travel in all directions. It's called a ripple effect. That's the kind of impact Christians are meant to have in this world—the kind of impact that the RHEMA family is producing in the earth today.

The Word Partner Club links Christians with a shared interest in reaching people with the Gospel and the message of faith in God.

Together we are reaching across generations, cultures, and nations to spread the Good News of Jesus Christ to every corner of the earth.

To join us in reaching the world,
visit **www.rhema.org/wpc** or call 1-866-312-0972.

Always on.

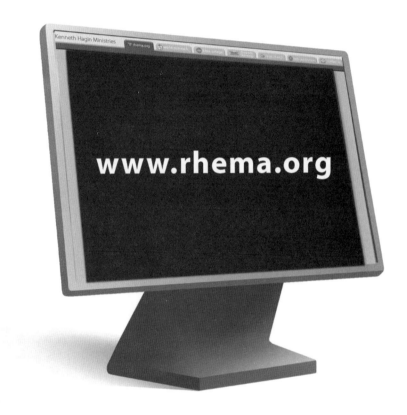

For the latest news and information on products, media, podcasts, study resources, and special offers, visit us online 24 hours a day.

www.rhema.org

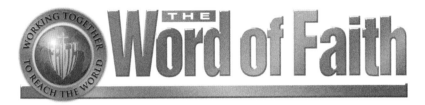

Free Subscription!

Call now to receive a free subscription to *The Word of Faith* magazine from Kenneth Hagin Ministries. Receive encouragement and spiritual refreshment from . . .

- *Faith-building articles from Kenneth W. Hagin, Lynette Hagin, and others*
- *"Timeless Teaching" from the archives of Kenneth E. Hagin*
- *Feature articles on prayer and healing*
- *Testimonies of salvation, healing, and deliverance*
- *Children's activity page*
- *Updates on RHEMA Bible Training Center, RHEMA Bible Church, and other outreaches of Kenneth Hagin Ministries*

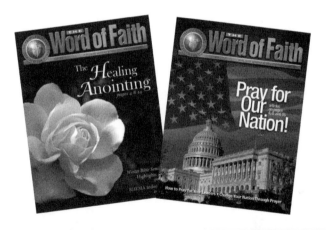

Subscribe today for your free *Word of Faith*!

1-888-28-FAITH (1-888-283-2484)

www.rhema.org/wof

OFFER CODE—BKORD:WF